BEYOND BLOOD SUGAR: EAT WELL, LIVE WELL

BY

DR. HELEN PAUL

DR. Helen Paul

668 Half and Half Drive, FRESNO

CA 93711

This Book is Dedicated to my beloved wife and child,

Your unwavering love and support have been my rock through every chapter of life. This book is dedicated to you, my pillars of strength and inspiration

Table Of Content

Chapter 1: Understanding

Diabetes and Diet

What is Diabetes?

Diabetes is a chronic health condition characterized by high levels of sugar (glucose) in the blood. This occurs when the body either does not produce enough insulin (a hormone that helps regulate blood sugar) or cannot effectively use the insulin it produces. Insulin is essential for allowing glucose to enter the body's cells, where it is used for energy. When insulin function is impaired, glucose builds up in the bloodstream, leading to high blood sugar levels.

Types of Diabetes

There are several types of diabetes, including:

1. Type 1 Diabetes: This type of diabetes occurs when the immune system mistakenly attacks and destroys the insulin-producing cells in the pancreas. As a result, the body is unable to produce insulin. Type 1 diabetes is typically diagnosed in children and young adults, although it can develop at any age. People with type 1 diabetes require insulin therapy to survive.

2. Type 2 Diabetes: Type 2 diabetes is the most common form of diabetes, accounting for the majority of diabetes cases worldwide. In type 2 diabetes, the body either does not produce enough insulin or becomes resistant to its effects. This leads to elevated blood sugar levels. Type 2 diabetes is often associated with lifestyle factors such as obesity, physical inactivity, and poor diet, although genetic and environmental factors also play a role.

3. Gestational Diabetes: Gestational diabetes occurs during pregnancy when the body is unable to produce enough insulin to meet the increased demands of

pregnancy. This can lead to high blood sugar levels, which can affect both the mother and the baby. Gestational diabetes typically resolves after childbirth, but women who have had gestational diabetes are at increased risk of developing type 2 diabetes later in life.

4. Other Types of Diabetes: There are other less common forms of diabetes, such as monogenic diabetes and secondary diabetes, which have different causes and characteristics.

- The Role of Diet in Diabetes Management

Diet plays a crucial role in managing diabetes and can significantly impact blood sugar levels, overall health, and quality of life for individuals with diabetes. The foods we eat directly affect our body's ability to regulate blood sugar levels, which is especially important for people with diabetes who need to carefully monitor and control their blood glucose levels.

1. Impact of Carbohydrates: Carbohydrates have the most direct effect on blood sugar levels because they are broken down into glucose during digestion. Therefore, managing carbohydrate intake is a key aspect of diabetes meal planning. Foods high in carbohydrates, such as bread, pasta, rice, and sugary snacks, can cause blood sugar levels to rise rapidly, while high-fiber carbohydrates, such as whole grains, fruits, and vegetables, are digested more slowly and have a gentler effect on blood sugar.

2. Balancing Macronutrients: In addition to carbohydrates, proteins and fats also play a role in diabetes management. Including lean proteins and healthy fats in meals can help slow down the digestion of carbohydrates, leading to more stable blood sugar levels after meals. Balancing macronutrients can also help control hunger and prevent overeating, which is important for managing weight and blood sugar levels.

3. Meal Timing and Frequency: The timing and frequency of meals can impact blood sugar control. Eating regular meals and snacks spaced throughout the day can help prevent large fluctuations in blood

sugar levels. Consistency in meal timing can also be beneficial, as it allows for more predictable insulin dosing and better overall blood sugar management.

4. Individualized Approach: It's important to recognize that there is no one-size-fits-all diet for diabetes. Each person's nutritional needs and preferences are unique, and dietary recommendations should be tailored to individual needs, taking into account factors such as age, activity level, medication regimen, and personal health goals.

5. Importance of Monitoring: Monitoring blood sugar levels regularly can provide valuable information about how different foods and meals affect blood sugar. This information can be used to make informed choices about food and to adjust meal plans as needed to achieve optimal blood sugar control.

Key dietary considerations for

diabetes:

1. Carbohydrate Intake: Carbohydrates have the most significant impact on blood sugar levels. Managing carbohydrate intake is crucial for people with diabetes. Focus on complex carbohydrates with a low glycemic index (GI), such as whole grains, legumes, and vegetables, which have a slower effect on blood sugar levels.

2. Portion Control: Controlling portion sizes helps manage calorie intake and prevents spikes in blood sugar levels. Use measuring cups or visual cues to estimate portion sizes and avoid overeating.

3. Balanced Meals: Aim for balanced meals that include a variety of food groups, including lean proteins, healthy fats, fiber-rich carbohydrates, and vegetables. This helps provide essential nutrients and prevents rapid fluctuations in blood sugar levels.

4. Fiber-Rich Foods: Fiber helps regulate blood sugar levels and improves digestive health. Incorporate fiber-rich foods like fruits, vegetables, whole grains, legumes, nuts, and seeds into your diet.

5. Healthy Fats: Choose healthy fats, such as those found in avocados, nuts, seeds, and olive oil, over saturated and trans fats. Healthy fats are important for heart health and can help improve insulin sensitivity.

6. Sugar and Sweeteners: Limit added sugars and sugary beverages, as they can cause rapid spikes in blood sugar levels. Use natural sweeteners like stevia or monk fruit in moderation if needed.

7. Meal Timing: Consistent meal timing can help regulate blood sugar levels. Aim for regular meals and snacks spaced throughout the day to prevent extreme fluctuations in blood sugar.

8. Hydration: Stay hydrated with water or other non-caloric beverages. Avoid sugary drinks and excessive caffeine, which can affect blood sugar levels and hydration status.

9. Alcohol Moderation: If you choose to drink alcohol, do so in moderation and with food. Alcohol can affect blood sugar levels and may interact with diabetes medications.

10. Individualized Approach: Work with a healthcare provider or registered dietitian to develop a personalized meal plan that considers your individual health goals, preferences, and lifestyle.

Chapter 2: Foundations of a Diabetes-Friendly Diet

Understanding Carbohydrates, Proteins, and Fats

Carbohydrates:
Carbohydrates are the body's primary source of energy and have a significant impact on blood sugar levels. They are found in foods like bread, rice, pasta, fruits, vegetables, and dairy products. Carbohydrates are broken down into glucose (sugar) during digestion, which is then used by the body for energy. However, people with diabetes need to be mindful of their carbohydrate intake to manage blood sugar levels effectively.

Proteins:

Proteins are essential for building and repairing tissues, and they play a role in many bodily functions. Foods rich in protein include meat, poultry, fish, eggs, dairy products, legumes, nuts, and seeds. Unlike carbohydrates, proteins have minimal impact on blood sugar levels and can help promote satiety and stabilize blood sugar when consumed as part of a balanced meal.

Fats:

Fats are an important source of energy and are necessary for the absorption of fat-soluble vitamins (A, D, E, and K) and the production of hormones. There are different types of fats, including saturated fats, trans fats, monounsaturated fats, and polyunsaturated fats. While some fats, such as saturated and trans fats, can increase the risk of heart disease and should be limited, others, like monounsaturated and polyunsaturated fats, are considered heart-healthy and can be included in a diabetes-friendly diet in moderation.

Balancing Carbohydrates, Proteins, and Fats:

A balanced meal for someone with diabetes includes a combination of carbohydrates, proteins, and fats. The

goal is to achieve a balance that helps stabilize blood sugar levels and provides essential nutrients. Some tips for balancing these macronutrients include:
- Prioritizing complex carbohydrates with a low glycemic index (GI) to minimize blood sugar spikes.
- Including lean sources of protein, such as poultry, fish, tofu, legumes, and low-fat dairy products.
- Choosing healthy fats, such as those found in avocados, nuts, seeds, and olive oil, while limiting saturated and trans fats.

The Importance of Fiber

Fiber is an essential component of a diabetes-friendly diet due to its many health benefits, particularly its impact on blood sugar levels, digestion, and heart health.

1. Blood Sugar Management: Fiber slows down the digestion and absorption of carbohydrates, which helps prevent rapid spikes in blood sugar levels after meals. Foods high in fiber have a lower glycemic index (GI), which means they have a less significant impact on blood sugar levels compared to low-fiber foods.

2. Improved Satiety: High-fiber foods are often more filling and can help promote a feeling of fullness, which may aid in weight management and portion control. This can be beneficial for individuals with diabetes who are working to achieve or maintain a healthy weight.

3. Digestive Health: Fiber plays a crucial role in maintaining a healthy digestive system. It adds bulk to stool, which can help prevent constipation and promote regular bowel movements. Additionally, some types of fiber, known as prebiotics, can support the growth of beneficial gut bacteria, which contribute to overall digestive health.

4. Heart Health: Fiber-rich diets have been associated with a reduced risk of heart disease. Soluble fiber, in particular, has been shown to help lower cholesterol levels, which can benefit heart health. Since individuals with diabetes are at an increased risk of heart disease, including fiber in the diet is especially important for managing overall cardiovascular health.

5. Food Sources of Fiber: Good sources of fiber include fruits, vegetables, whole grains, legumes

(beans, lentils), nuts, and seeds. Aim to include a variety of these foods in your diet to ensure you're getting an adequate intake of fiber.

6. Recommendations: The Dietary Guidelines for Americans recommend a daily fiber intake of 25 grams for women and 38 grams for men. However, individual fiber needs may vary based on factors such as age, sex, and overall health.

Glycemic Index and Glycemic Load

The glycemic index (GI) and glycemic load (GL) are two important concepts related to carbohydrate-containing foods and their impact on blood sugar levels. Understanding these concepts can help individuals with diabetes make informed choices about the foods they eat.

1. Glycemic Index (GI): The GI is a measure of how quickly a carbohydrate-containing food raises blood sugar levels after consumption compared to pure glucose, which has a GI of 100. Foods with a high GI (above 70) are rapidly digested and cause a rapid

increase in blood sugar levels, while foods with a low GI (below 55) are digested more slowly and cause a slower, more gradual increase in blood sugar levels.

2. Glycemic Load (GL): The glycemic load takes into account both the GI of a food and the amount of carbohydrates it contains per serving. It provides a more accurate picture of how a food affects blood sugar levels than the GI alone. Foods with a high GL may cause a larger spike in blood sugar levels, especially if consumed in large quantities, while foods with a low GL have a smaller impact on blood sugar levels.

3. Using GI and GL for Meal Planning: For individuals with diabetes, choosing foods with a lower GI and GL can help prevent rapid spikes in blood sugar levels. Foods with a lower GI and GL are generally more slowly digested and can help provide a more steady release of energy. Examples of low-GI foods include most non-starchy vegetables, legumes, whole grains, nuts, and seeds. Foods with a higher GI, such as white bread, sugary cereals, and processed snacks, should be consumed in moderation or avoided.

4. Limitations of GI and GL: While the GI and GL can be useful tools for meal planning, they are not the only factors to consider. The overall nutrient content of a food, portion size, and the combination of foods eaten together can also influence how it affects blood sugar levels. It's important to consider these factors in the context of an overall healthy eating pattern.

Portion Control and Meal Planning

1. Importance of Portion Control: Controlling portion sizes is essential for managing blood sugar levels and maintaining a healthy weight. Large portions can lead to overeating, which can cause spikes in blood sugar and contribute to weight gain. Learning to estimate portion sizes and practicing mindful eating can help prevent overconsumption.

2. Tips for Portion Control:
   - Use smaller plates and bowls to visually reduce portion sizes.
   - Measure portions using standard kitchen tools, such as measuring cups and spoons.

- Pay attention to serving sizes on food labels to avoid consuming more than recommended.
- Be mindful of portion distortion when dining out, as restaurant servings are often larger than necessary.

3. Meal Planning Strategies:
- Plan meals ahead of time to ensure balanced and nutritious choices.
- Include a variety of foods from different food groups, such as lean proteins, whole grains, vegetables, and healthy fats, in each meal.
- Aim for balanced meals that provide a mix of carbohydrates, proteins, and fats to help regulate blood sugar levels and provide sustained energy.
- Consider the glycemic index (GI) of foods when planning meals. Choosing lower GI foods can help prevent rapid spikes in blood sugar.

4. Importance of Consistency: Consistency in meal timing and portion sizes can help regulate blood sugar levels and prevent extreme fluctuations. Try to eat meals and snacks at regular intervals throughout the day to maintain steady energy levels.

5. Meal Planning Tools:

- Use meal planning apps or tools to help organize and plan meals.
- Consider using a food diary or journal to track meals, portion sizes, and blood sugar levels to identify patterns and make adjustments as needed.

6. Flexibility and Adaptability: While meal planning is important, it's also essential to be flexible and adaptable. Life can be unpredictable, and being able to adjust your meal plan when necessary can help you stay on track with your diabetes management goals.

7. Consulting a Registered Dietitian: For personalized meal planning guidance tailored to your specific needs and preferences, consider consulting a registered dietitian with experience in diabetes management. They can provide individualized meal plans and practical tips to help you achieve your dietary goals.

Chapter 3: Carbohydrate

Counting and Meal Planning

Carbohydrate Counting Basics

1. Understanding Carbohydrates: Carbohydrates are one of the main nutrients in food and have the most significant impact on blood sugar levels. They are found in a wide variety of foods, including grains, fruits, vegetables, dairy products, and sweets. Carbohydrates are broken down into glucose (sugar) in the body, which is used for energy.

2. Role of Carbohydrates in Blood Sugar Management: For individuals with diabetes, monitoring carbohydrate intake is crucial for managing blood sugar levels. Different carbohydrates affect blood sugar levels differently, so it's important to

understand the concept of glycemic index (GI) and glycemic load (GL). Foods with a lower GI and GL are less likely to cause rapid spikes in blood sugar levels.

3. Carbohydrate Counting Method: Carbohydrate counting is a meal planning approach that involves tracking the amount of carbohydrates consumed in meals and snacks. It allows for flexibility in food choices while helping to maintain consistent blood sugar levels.

4. How to Count Carbohydrates:
  - Identify carbohydrate-containing foods in your meals and snacks, including grains, starchy vegetables, fruits, dairy products, and sweets.
  - Learn to estimate portion sizes and the carbohydrate content of common foods. Food labels can provide valuable information about carbohydrate content per serving.
  - Use tools such as carbohydrate counting apps, food scales, or measuring cups and spoons to help you accurately measure and track carbohydrate intake.
  - Monitor your blood sugar levels regularly to see how different foods and portions affect your blood sugar.

5. Setting Carbohydrate Goals: Work with a healthcare provider or registered dietitian to determine your daily carbohydrate goals based on factors such as your age, weight, activity level, and blood sugar targets. Your goals may need to be adjusted over time based on changes in your health or medication regimen.

6. Flexibility and Variety: Carbohydrate counting offers flexibility in food choices, allowing you to include a variety of foods in your meals and snacks. It can be adapted to different cultural preferences and dietary needs.

7. Meal Planning with Carbohydrate Counting: Use your carbohydrate goals to plan balanced meals that include a mix of carbohydrates, proteins, and fats. Consider the timing of your meals and snacks to help manage blood sugar levels throughout the day.

Sample Meal Plans for Different Calorie Levels

When planning meals for diabetes management, it's important to consider individual calorie needs based on factors such as age, gender, weight, activity level, and metabolic rate. Below are sample meal plans for different calorie levels that can be adjusted to suit individual needs. These meal plans focus on carbohydrate counting and portion control while providing balanced nutrition.

Note: The following meal plans are for illustrative purposes only and should be adjusted based on individual dietary requirements and preferences. It's important to consult with a healthcare provider or registered dietitian for personalized meal planning.

Sample Meal Plan for 1,500 Calories

- Breakfast:
  - 1 small whole-grain English muffin
  - 1 tablespoon of peanut butter

  - 1 small apple

  - 1 cup of unsweetened almond milk

- Snack:

  - 10 baby carrots

  - 2 tablespoons of hummus

- Lunch:

  - Grilled chicken breast (3 oz)

  - Mixed green salad with cherry tomatoes, cucumber,
and balsamic vinaigrette

  - 1 small whole-grain roll

- Snack:

  - Greek yogurt (6 oz) with a handful of mixed berries

- Dinner:

  - Baked salmon fillet (4 oz)

  - Steamed broccoli

  - 1/2 cup of quinoa

Sample Meal Plan for 1,600 Calories

- Breakfast:

  - 1 small whole-grain bagel with cream cheese

  - 1 boiled egg

- 1 medium orange
  - 1 cup of green tea

- Snack:
  - 1/2 cup of cottage cheese
  - 1/2 cup of pineapple chunks

- Lunch:
  - Tuna salad made with canned tuna, mixed greens, cherry tomatoes, cucumber, and vinaigrette
  - 1 small whole-grain roll

- Snack:
  - 1 ounce of almonds
  - 1 small apple

- Dinner:
  - Baked cod fillet (4 oz)
  - Steamed broccoli
  - 1/2 cup of quinoa

Sample Meal Plan for 1,800 Calories

- Breakfast:
  - Greek yogurt (6 oz) with a handful of mixed berries

  - 1 slice of whole-grain toast with almond butter

  - 1 small banana

  - 1 cup of herbal tea

- Snack:

  - 1 small orange

  - 10 baby carrots with hummus

- Lunch:

  - Grilled chicken Caesar salad with romaine lettuce, grilled chicken breast, cherry tomatoes, Parmesan cheese, and Caesar dressing

  - 1 small whole-grain roll

- Snack:

  - 1/2 cup of low-fat cottage cheese

  - 1/2 cup of pineapple chunks

- Dinner:

  - Stir-fried tofu with mixed vegetables (bell peppers, broccoli, carrots) served with brown rice

  - 1 small apple

Sample Meal Plan for 2,000 Calories

- Breakfast:
  - 2 slices of whole-grain toast
  - 2 tablespoons of almond butter
  - 1 banana
  - 1 cup of unsweetened soy milk

- Snack:
  - 1 small orange
  - 1 ounce of almonds

- Lunch:
  - Turkey and avocado wrap with whole-grain tortilla
  - Mixed green salad with vinaigrette
  - 1 small apple

- Snack:
  - 1/2 cup of cottage cheese with pineapple chunks

- Dinner:
  - Grilled sirloin steak (5 oz)
  - Roasted sweet potatoes
  - Steamed green beans

Sample Meal Plan for 2,200 Calories

- Breakfast:

- Scrambled eggs (2 eggs) with spinach and feta cheese
  - 2 slices of whole-grain toast with avocado
  - 1 medium orange
  - 1 cup of skim milk

- Snack:
  - 1 ounce of mixed nuts
  - 1/2 cup of mixed berries

- Lunch:
  - Grilled salmon fillet (5 oz)
  - Quinoa salad with mixed vegetables (cucumbers, cherry tomatoes, red onion) and vinaigrette dressing
  - 1 small pear

- Snack:
  - 1 cup of low-fat yogurt with sliced banana

- Dinner:
  - Turkey chili made with lean ground turkey, kidney beans, tomatoes, and spices
  - 1 small whole-grain roll

Sample Meal Plan for 2,500 Calories

- Breakfast:
  - Vegetable omelet made with 2 eggs, spinach, and bell peppers
  - 2 slices of whole-grain toast
  - 1 small orange
  - 1 cup of skim milk

- Snack:
  - 1 ounce of mixed nuts
  - 1/2 cup of mixed berries

- Lunch:
  - Quinoa salad with mixed vegetables, chickpeas, and feta cheese
  - Whole-grain roll
  - 1 small pear

- Snack:
  - 1 cup of low-fat yogurt with sliced banana

- Dinner:
  - Grilled chicken breast (6 oz)
  - Brown rice pilaf
  - Steamed asparagus

Tips for Dining Out with Diabetes

Dining out can present challenges for individuals with diabetes, but with careful planning and mindful choices, it is possible to enjoy meals while managing blood sugar levels effectively. Here are some tips for dining out with diabetes:

1. Research the Restaurant: Before dining out, research the restaurant's menu online or call ahead to inquire about the availability of diabetes-friendly options. Look for restaurants that offer a variety of healthy choices, such as grilled proteins, salads, and vegetable sides.

2. Choose Wisely: When reviewing the menu, focus on selecting balanced meals that include lean proteins, vegetables, and whole grains. Avoid dishes that are high in refined carbohydrates, saturated fats, and added sugars.

3. Portion Control: Pay attention to portion sizes, which can be larger than necessary in restaurants. Consider sharing a meal with a dining companion or

asking for a half-portion if available. Avoid all-you-can-eat buffets, as they can lead to overeating.

4. Ask Questions: Don't hesitate to ask your server about how dishes are prepared and whether modifications can be made to accommodate your dietary needs. Requesting sauces and dressings on the side can help you control your intake of added sugars and fats.

5. Be Mindful of Beverages: Choose beverages without added sugars, such as water, unsweetened tea, or sparkling water. Avoid sugary sodas, fruit juices, and alcoholic beverages with high sugar content.

6. Control Your Sides: Opt for healthier side options, such as steamed vegetables or a side salad with vinaigrette dressing, instead of fried foods or dishes with heavy sauces.

7. Watch for Hidden Sugars: Be mindful of hidden sugars in sauces, dressings, and marinades. These can contribute to a higher carbohydrate content in your meal.

8. Monitor Your Blood Sugar: Check your blood sugar before and after dining out to monitor how your meal choices affect your levels. This can help you make adjustments to your meal plan as needed.

9. Plan Ahead for Special Occasions: For special occasions or planned dining out experiences, adjust your meal plan and medication as necessary in consultation with your healthcare provider.

10. Enjoy in Moderation: While it's important to make healthy choices, it's also okay to enjoy a treat occasionally. Just be mindful of portion sizes and overall balance in your diet.

Chapter 4: Managing Blood

Sugar Levels with Food

Foods That Affect Blood Sugar

Levels

Understanding how different foods impact blood sugar levels is essential for managing diabetes effectively. Here are some key points about foods that affect blood sugar levels:

1. Carbohydrates: Carbohydrates have the most significant impact on blood sugar levels because they are broken down into glucose (sugar) during digestion. Foods high in carbohydrates include grains, starchy vegetables (like potatoes and corn), fruits, dairy products, and sweets. It's important to be

mindful of portion sizes and choose complex carbohydrates, which are digested more slowly and have a less dramatic effect on blood sugar levels than simple carbohydrates.

2. Proteins: Proteins have a minimal impact on blood sugar levels because they are not converted into glucose as quickly as carbohydrates. However, large amounts of protein can affect blood sugar levels if consumed in excess. Choose lean sources of protein, such as poultry, fish, tofu, legumes, and nuts, and be mindful of portion sizes.

3. Fats: Fats have little direct effect on blood sugar levels. However, foods high in unhealthy fats, such as saturated and trans fats, can contribute to insulin resistance and increase the risk of heart disease, which is a concern for people with diabetes. Choose healthy fats, such as those found in avocados, nuts, seeds, and olive oil, in moderation.

4. Fiber: Fiber is a type of carbohydrate that is not fully digested by the body. It can help regulate blood sugar levels by slowing the absorption of glucose and improving insulin sensitivity. Foods high in fiber include fruits, vegetables, whole grains, legumes, nuts,

and seeds. Aim to include a variety of high-fiber foods in your diet.

5. Glycemic Index (GI): The glycemic index is a measure of how quickly a carbohydrate-containing food raises blood sugar levels. Foods with a high GI (such as white bread and sugary cereals) cause a rapid spike in blood sugar, while foods with a low GI (like whole grains and legumes) cause a slower, more gradual rise in blood sugar. Choosing lower GI foods can help stabilize blood sugar levels.

6. Timing and Balance: The timing and balance of meals and snacks can also impact blood sugar levels. Eating regular, balanced meals and snacks throughout the day can help prevent extreme fluctuations in blood sugar levels.

Understanding the Role of Insulin

Insulin is a hormone produced by the pancreas that plays a crucial role in regulating blood sugar levels. Its primary function is to facilitate the uptake of glucose from the bloodstream into cells, where it can be used for energy or stored for future use. In individuals with diabetes, there may be insufficient insulin production or an inability of the body to use insulin effectively, leading to elevated blood sugar levels.

Key points about the role of insulin in managing blood sugar levels with food include:

1. Carbohydrate Metabolism: When you eat carbohydrates, they are broken down into glucose, which enters the bloodstream. In response, the pancreas releases insulin to help transport glucose into cells, thereby lowering blood sugar levels.

2. Insulin Resistance: In type 2 diabetes, cells become resistant to the effects of insulin, leading to elevated blood sugar levels. This can result in the pancreas producing more insulin in an attempt to compensate, which can further contribute to insulin resistance over time.

3. Meal Timing and Insulin: The timing of meals can impact insulin requirements. Eating carbohydrates causes a rise in blood sugar, which triggers the release of insulin. Understanding how different foods affect

blood sugar levels can help you time your meals and insulin doses effectively.

4. Insulin Therapy: For individuals with type 1 diabetes or advanced type 2 diabetes, insulin therapy may be necessary to manage blood sugar levels. Insulin can be administered through injections or an insulin pump to mimic the body's natural insulin production.

5. Adjusting Insulin Doses: The amount of insulin needed can vary based on factors such as meal composition, physical activity, stress, illness, and individual insulin sensitivity. It's important to work with a healthcare provider to determine the appropriate insulin regimen and make adjustments as needed.

6. Meal Planning and Insulin: When planning meals, consider the timing and composition of your meals in relation to your insulin doses. This can help you match your insulin levels to your carbohydrate intake and prevent blood sugar fluctuations.

7. Monitoring Blood Sugar Levels: Regularly monitoring your blood sugar levels can help you understand how different foods and insulin doses

affect your blood sugar. This information can guide your meal planning and insulin management.

8. Consistency and Balance: Consistent meal timing, portion control, and a balanced diet can help maintain stable blood sugar levels and reduce the need for large insulin doses.

Strategies for Stabilizing Blood Sugar Levels

1. Focus on Whole Foods: Base your diet on whole, unprocessed foods such as vegetables, fruits, whole grains, lean proteins, and healthy fats. These foods are rich in nutrients and fiber, which can help stabilize blood sugar levels.

2. Choose Low-Glycemic Index Foods: Foods with a low glycemic index (GI) are digested more slowly, leading to a gradual rise in blood sugar levels. Examples include legumes, non-starchy vegetables, whole grains, and most fruits.

3. Monitor Carbohydrate Intake: Carbohydrates have the most significant impact on blood sugar levels. Carbohydrate counting can help you manage your intake and prevent spikes in blood sugar. Consider working with a dietitian to learn how to count carbohydrates effectively.

4. Eat Regular Meals and Snacks: Eating regular meals and snacks spaced throughout the day can help prevent extreme fluctuations in blood sugar levels. Aim for balanced meals that include a mix of carbohydrates, proteins, and fats.

5. Include Protein with Each Meal: Protein can help slow down the digestion of carbohydrates, leading to a more gradual rise in blood sugar levels. Include sources of lean protein such as poultry, fish, tofu, beans, and legumes with each meal.

6. Choose Healthy Fats: Healthy fats, such as those found in avocados, nuts, seeds, and olive oil, can help improve insulin sensitivity and stabilize blood sugar levels. Limit saturated and trans fats found in processed and fried foods.

7. Fiber-Rich Foods: Fiber slows down the absorption of sugar into the bloodstream and can help improve blood sugar control. Include plenty of fiber-rich foods such as vegetables, fruits, whole grains, legumes, nuts, and seeds in your diet.

8. Stay Hydrated: Drink plenty of water throughout the day to stay hydrated. Dehydration can affect blood sugar levels, so it's essential to maintain adequate fluid intake.

9. Avoid Sugary Beverages and Snacks: Sugary beverages and snacks can cause rapid spikes in blood sugar levels. Choose water, unsweetened tea, or other non-caloric beverages, and opt for healthier snack options such as nuts, seeds, or vegetables with hummus.

10. Monitor Your Blood Sugar: Regularly monitor your blood sugar levels to track how different foods and meals affect your levels. This can help you make informed choices and adjust your diet as needed to maintain stable blood sugar levels.

The Impact of Alcohol on Blood

Sugar

Alcohol can affect blood sugar levels in several ways, and it's important for individuals with diabetes to be mindful of its impact when consuming alcoholic beverages. Here are some key points to consider regarding alcohol and blood sugar:

1. Hypoglycemia Risk: Alcohol can lower blood sugar levels, especially if consumed on an empty stomach or in large quantities. This can increase the risk of hypoglycemia (low blood sugar) for individuals taking insulin or certain diabetes medications that lower blood sugar.

2. Delayed Hypoglycemia: While alcohol initially lowers blood sugar levels, it can lead to delayed hypoglycemia several hours after consumption. This delayed effect can make it challenging to predict and manage blood sugar levels.

3. Carbohydrate Content: Alcoholic beverages contain varying amounts of carbohydrates, which can impact blood sugar levels. Sweetened drinks, such as cocktails and mixed drinks, can have a higher carbohydrate content and raise blood sugar levels more than other types of alcohol.

4. Timing and Moderation: If you choose to consume alcohol, do so in moderation and with food. Eating a meal or snack containing carbohydrates before drinking can help mitigate the risk of hypoglycemia.

5. Monitoring Blood Sugar: Check your blood sugar levels before, during, and after consuming alcohol to monitor its impact on your levels. Be prepared to take appropriate action if your blood sugar levels become too high or too low.

6. Alcohol and Medications: Some diabetes medications, particularly those that stimulate insulin production or increase insulin sensitivity, can interact with alcohol and affect blood sugar levels. Consult your healthcare provider to understand how alcohol may interact with your specific medications.

7. Alcohol and Weight Management: Alcoholic beverages are often high in calories and can contribute to weight gain if consumed in excess. Managing weight is an important aspect of diabetes management, so it's important to be mindful of the calorie content of alcoholic drinks.

8. Choosing Wisely: Opt for lower-carbohydrate and lower-calorie alcoholic beverages, such as light beer or dry wines, when possible. Avoid sugary mixers and high-calorie cocktails.

9. Know Your Limits: Be aware of your personal tolerance for alcohol and how it affects your blood sugar levels. Everyone's response to alcohol can be different, so it's important to know your limits and drink responsibly.

Chapter 5: The Role of

Protein and Fats in Diabetes

Choosing Healthy Sources of

Protein

Protein is an essential nutrient that plays a crucial role in the body's growth, repair, and maintenance. When it comes to managing diabetes, choosing healthy sources of protein is important for maintaining blood sugar levels and overall health. Here are some tips for selecting healthy sources of protein:

1. Lean Protein Choices: Opt for lean sources of protein, such as skinless poultry, fish, tofu, tempeh, legumes (beans, lentils), and low-fat dairy products (yogurt, milk, cheese). These options are lower in

saturated fat and calories compared to fatty cuts of meat.

2. Plant-Based Proteins: Incorporate plant-based protein sources into your diet, such as beans, lentils, chickpeas, quinoa, nuts, and seeds. These foods are rich in fiber, which can help regulate blood sugar levels and improve satiety.

3. Fatty Fish: Include fatty fish, such as salmon, mackerel, sardines, and trout, in your diet. These fish are high in omega-3 fatty acids, which have anti-inflammatory properties and are beneficial for heart health.

4. Limit Processed Meats: Limit consumption of processed meats, such as bacon, sausage, hot dogs, and deli meats, which are high in sodium and saturated fat. These meats have been associated with an increased risk of heart disease and other health issues.

5. Portion Control: Pay attention to portion sizes when consuming protein-rich foods. Aim to include a moderate amount of protein in each meal, as excessive protein intake can contribute to weight gain

and may have negative effects on kidney function in some individuals with diabetes.

6. Preparation Methods: Choose healthy cooking methods, such as grilling, baking, steaming, or broiling, to prepare protein-rich foods. Avoid frying or cooking with excessive amounts of added fats, which can increase calorie and fat intake.

7. Reading Labels: When purchasing packaged foods, read the nutrition labels to check for the protein content, as well as the presence of added sugars, sodium, and unhealthy fats.

8. Balanced Meals: Incorporate a balance of protein, carbohydrates, and healthy fats into your meals to help maintain stable blood sugar levels and promote overall health.

Incorporating Healthy Fats into

Your Diet

Healthy fats play a crucial role in a balanced diet for individuals with diabetes. While it's important to moderate fat intake, choosing the right types of fats can have positive effects on overall health and blood sugar management. Here's how to incorporate healthy fats into your diet:

1. Choose Unsaturated Fats: Unsaturated fats, including monounsaturated and polyunsaturated fats, are considered heart-healthy and can help improve insulin sensitivity. Sources of unsaturated fats include:
  - Olive oil
  - Avocados
  - Nuts (almonds, walnuts, cashews)
  - Seeds (flaxseeds, chia seeds, sunflower seeds)
  - Fatty fish (salmon, mackerel, sardines)

2. Limit Saturated and Trans Fats: Saturated and trans fats can raise LDL cholesterol levels and increase the

risk of heart disease. Limit intake of foods high in these fats, such as:
  - Red meat
  - Full-fat dairy products
  - Processed foods (cakes, cookies, pastries) containing hydrogenated oils

3. Cook with Healthy Oils: Use heart-healthy oils like olive oil, canola oil, and avocado oil for cooking and salad dressings. These oils are rich in monounsaturated fats and can be part of a healthy diet for diabetes management.

4. Add Omega-3 Fatty Acids: Omega-3 fatty acids, found in fatty fish, flaxseeds, and walnuts, have anti-inflammatory properties and may help reduce the risk of heart disease. Consider incorporating sources of omega-3s into your diet regularly.

5. Read Food Labels: When choosing packaged foods, check the nutrition labels for the type and amount of fats they contain. Look for products with lower saturated and trans fat content.

6. Be Mindful of Portions: While healthy fats are beneficial, they are calorie-dense. Be mindful of

portion sizes to avoid excess calorie intake, which can contribute to weight gain.

7. Balance with Other Nutrients: Incorporate healthy fats into balanced meals that also include lean proteins, complex carbohydrates, and fiber-rich foods. This helps create satisfying meals that can help stabilize blood sugar levels.

8. Work with a Dietitian: If you're unsure how to incorporate healthy fats into your diet or need personalized guidance, consider consulting a registered dietitian. They can provide individualized recommendations based on your dietary preferences and health goals.

Chapter 6: The Importance of Fiber and Micronutrients

Benefits of Dietary Fiber for Diabetes

Dietary fiber plays a crucial role in the management of diabetes and overall health. It is a type of carbohydrate that the body cannot digest, and it comes in two main forms: soluble fiber and insoluble fiber. Both types of fiber offer various benefits for individuals with diabetes:

1. Blood Sugar Control: Soluble fiber can help stabilize blood sugar levels by slowing down the absorption of sugar into the bloodstream. This can prevent rapid

spikes in blood sugar after meals, which is especially beneficial for people with diabetes.

2. Improved Insulin Sensitivity: Some studies suggest that a high-fiber diet may improve insulin sensitivity, allowing the body to use insulin more effectively to regulate blood sugar levels. This can be particularly beneficial for individuals with type 2 diabetes.

3. Weight Management: High-fiber foods are often low in calories and can help you feel full and satisfied after meals, which may aid in weight management. Maintaining a healthy weight is important for managing diabetes and reducing the risk of complications.

4. Heart Health: Fiber-rich foods can help lower cholesterol levels and improve heart health. This is important for people with diabetes, as they have an increased risk of developing heart disease.

5. Digestive Health: Insoluble fiber adds bulk to the stool and can help promote regular bowel movements, preventing constipation. A healthy digestive system is essential for overall well-being.

6. Sources of Dietary Fiber: Good sources of dietary fiber include fruits, vegetables, whole grains, legumes, nuts, and seeds. Aim to include a variety of these foods in your diet to ensure an adequate intake of fiber.

7. Recommended Intake: The American Diabetes Association (ADA) recommends that adults with diabetes consume at least 25 to 30 grams of dietary fiber per day from food sources, rather than supplements. Gradually increase your fiber intake to avoid digestive discomfort.

8. Hydration: Drink plenty of water when increasing your fiber intake, as fiber absorbs water and can help prevent constipation. Adequate hydration is important for overall health, especially when consuming a high-fiber diet.

Sources of Dietary Fiber

Dietary fiber is an essential component of a healthy diet, especially for individuals with diabetes. It plays a crucial role in regulating blood sugar levels, promoting digestive health, and supporting overall well-being. Including a variety of fiber-rich foods in your diet can help you meet your nutritional needs and manage your diabetes more effectively. Here are some excellent sources of dietary fiber:

1. Whole Grains: Whole grains are rich in fiber, vitamins, and minerals. Choose whole grain options such as brown rice, quinoa, barley, oats, and whole wheat bread and pasta. These foods provide both soluble and insoluble fiber, which can help stabilize blood sugar levels and improve digestive health.

2. Legumes: Legumes, including beans, lentils, and peas, are excellent sources of fiber and protein. They are also low in fat and have a low glycemic index, making them a great choice for individuals with diabetes. Incorporate legumes into soups, salads, stews, and side dishes for added fiber and nutrition.

3. Fruits: Many fruits are rich in dietary fiber, particularly when eaten with the skin or pulp. Berries, apples, pears, oranges, and kiwi are good sources of fiber. Aim to include a variety of fruits in your diet to benefit from their fiber content and other essential nutrients.

4. Vegetables: Vegetables are high in fiber and low in calories, making them an ideal choice for diabetes management. Dark leafy greens, broccoli, Brussels sprouts, carrots, and sweet potatoes are examples of fiber-rich vegetables that can be enjoyed in salads, stir-fries, or as side dishes.

5. Nuts and Seeds: Nuts and seeds are nutrient-dense foods that provide fiber, healthy fats, and protein. Almonds, walnuts, chia seeds, flaxseeds, and pumpkin seeds are good options to incorporate into your diet for added fiber and micronutrients. However, be mindful of portion sizes due to their calorie density.

6. Whole Grain Cereals and Bread: Choose whole grain breakfast cereals and bread that are high in fiber and low in added sugars. Look for products that list whole grains as the first ingredient and have at least 3 grams of fiber per serving.

7. Fiber Supplements: In some cases, fiber supplements such as psyllium husk or methylcellulose may be recommended to increase fiber intake. However, it's best to obtain fiber from whole foods

whenever possible, as they provide a broader range of nutrients and health benefits.

Micronutrients Essential for

Diabetes Management

Micronutrients are essential vitamins and minerals that play a critical role in overall health and can be particularly important for individuals with diabetes. While they are required in smaller amounts compared to macronutrients (carbohydrates, proteins, and fats), micronutrients are vital for various bodily functions, including metabolism, immune function, and the maintenance of healthy tissues. Here are some key micronutrients that are especially important for diabetes management:

1. Vitamin D: Vitamin D plays a crucial role in calcium absorption and bone health. Low levels of vitamin D have been associated with an increased risk of type 2 diabetes and poor blood sugar control. Sources of vitamin D include sunlight exposure, fatty fish (such as

salmon and mackerel), fortified dairy products, and supplements.

2. Magnesium: Magnesium is involved in over 300 enzymatic reactions in the body, including those related to glucose metabolism and insulin sensitivity. Studies have suggested that magnesium deficiency may be associated with an increased risk of type 2 diabetes. Good food sources of magnesium include nuts, seeds, whole grains, leafy green vegetables, and legumes.

3. Chromium: Chromium is a mineral that has been studied for its potential role in improving insulin sensitivity and glucose metabolism. While more research is needed to fully understand its effects, some studies have suggested that chromium supplementation may benefit individuals with diabetes. Food sources of chromium include broccoli, grape juice, whole grains, and lean meats.

4. Omega-3 Fatty Acids: Omega-3 fatty acids, found primarily in fatty fish (such as salmon, mackerel, and sardines), flaxseeds, and walnuts, have been shown to have anti-inflammatory properties and may help reduce the risk of cardiovascular disease, which is

common in individuals with diabetes. They may also have a positive impact on insulin sensitivity.

5. B Vitamins: B vitamins, including B1 (thiamine), B6 (pyridoxine), and B12 (cobalamin), are important for nerve function, energy production, and the metabolism of carbohydrates, proteins, and fats. Some studies have suggested that individuals with diabetes may have an increased need for certain B vitamins. Good food sources of B vitamins include fortified cereals, whole grains, meat, fish, and leafy green vegetables.

6. Antioxidants: Antioxidants, such as vitamins C and E, and selenium, help protect cells from damage caused by free radicals and oxidative stress. Some research suggests that antioxidants may play a role in reducing the risk of complications associated with diabetes, such as cardiovascular disease. Foods rich in antioxidants include fruits, vegetables, nuts, seeds, and whole grains.

7. Zinc: Zinc is involved in numerous metabolic processes, including insulin storage and release. It also plays a role in immune function and wound healing, which can be particularly important for individuals

with diabetes. Good sources of zinc include oysters, red meat, poultry, beans, nuts, and whole grains.

8. Fiber: While not a micronutrient, dietary fiber is an essential component of a diabetes-friendly diet. Fiber helps regulate blood sugar levels, improve satiety, and support digestive health. It is found in plant foods such as fruits, vegetables, whole grains, nuts, and seeds.

Incorporating a variety of nutrient-dense foods that are rich in these micronutrients into your diet can help support your overall health and diabetes management. However, it's important to remember that individual nutrient needs can vary based on factors such as age, sex, health status, and medication use. Consulting with a registered dietitian or healthcare provider can help you determine your specific nutrient needs and develop a personalized nutrition plan tailored to your individual requirements.

Supplements and Their Role in

Diabetes Care

While a well-balanced diet rich in whole foods is the foundation of diabetes management, some individuals may benefit from dietary supplements to fill nutrient gaps or address specific health concerns. Here's a look at supplements and their potential role in diabetes care:

1. Vitamin and Mineral Supplements:
   - Certain vitamins and minerals play a crucial role in overall health and may be especially important for individuals with diabetes. These include vitamin D, magnesium, and chromium, among others.
   - Vitamin D: Adequate vitamin D levels are important for bone health and may also play a role in insulin sensitivity. Some studies suggest that low vitamin D levels are associated with an increased risk of developing type 2 diabetes.
   - Magnesium: Magnesium is involved in glucose metabolism and insulin action. Low magnesium levels

have been linked to insulin resistance and an increased risk of type 2 diabetes.

   - Chromium: Chromium is a trace mineral that may enhance the action of insulin and improve glucose tolerance. However, research on the effectiveness of chromium supplements for diabetes management is mixed.

2. Omega-3 Fatty Acids:

   - Omega-3 fatty acids, found in fish oil supplements, have anti-inflammatory properties and may benefit heart health. Some studies suggest that omega-3 fatty acids may also improve lipid profiles and reduce cardiovascular risk factors in individuals with diabetes.

3. Fiber Supplements:

   - Fiber is important for digestive health and can help regulate blood sugar levels. While it's best to obtain fiber from whole foods like fruits, vegetables, and whole grains, some individuals may benefit from fiber supplements, especially if their dietary fiber intake is inadequate.

4. Probiotics:

   - Probiotics are beneficial bacteria that can help maintain gut health. Some research suggests that probiotics may have a modest effect on blood sugar levels and insulin sensitivity in individuals with diabetes.

5. Herbal Supplements:

  - Some herbal supplements, such as cinnamon and fenugreek, have been studied for their potential benefits in diabetes management. However, more research is needed to determine their effectiveness and safety.

6. Considerations and Precautions:

  - Before taking any dietary supplement, it's important to consult with a healthcare provider, especially if you have diabetes or any other medical condition. Some supplements may interact with medications or have side effects.

  - It's best to obtain nutrients from whole foods whenever possible, as they contain a variety of beneficial compounds that may not be present in isolated supplements.

  - Supplements should complement, not replace, a healthy diet and lifestyle. They are not a substitute for proper nutrition and should be used in conjunction with a well-balanced diet and regular physical activity.

While supplements can potentially play a role in supporting overall health and diabetes management, they should be used judiciously and under the guidance of a healthcare provider to ensure safety and effectiveness.

Chapter 7: Special Considerations for Diabetes and Weight Management

Understanding Weight and Diabetes

Weight management is a key component of diabetes care, as excess body weight can contribute to insulin resistance and make it more challenging to manage blood sugar levels. Understanding the relationship between weight and diabetes is essential for effective diabetes management. Here are some important points to consider:

1. Body Weight and Insulin Sensitivity:
   - Excess body weight, especially abdominal fat, can lead to insulin resistance, where the body's cells become less responsive to insulin. This can result in higher blood sugar levels and an increased risk of developing type 2 diabetes.
   - Losing even a modest amount of weight (5-10% of body weight) can improve insulin sensitivity and glycemic control in individuals with diabetes.

2. Weight and Diabetes Complications:
   - Maintaining a healthy weight is important for reducing the risk of diabetes-related complications, such as heart disease, stroke, kidney disease, and nerve damage.
   - Excess body weight can also contribute to other health issues commonly associated with diabetes, such as high blood pressure and high cholesterol levels.

3. Weight Loss Strategies:

- For individuals with diabetes who are overweight or obese, weight loss can significantly improve diabetes management and overall health.

- Strategies for weight loss typically include a combination of dietary changes, increased physical activity, and behavior modification.

- Aiming for gradual, sustainable weight loss of 1-2 pounds per week is generally recommended to achieve long-term success.

4. Importance of Diet and Physical Activity:

- A healthy diet and regular physical activity are key components of any weight management plan for individuals with diabetes.

- A balanced diet that is rich in fruits, vegetables, whole grains, lean proteins, and healthy fats can support weight loss and improve blood sugar control.

- Regular physical activity helps burn calories, improve insulin sensitivity, and maintain muscle mass, all of which are beneficial for weight management and diabetes care.

5. Monitoring and Support:

- Regular monitoring of weight, blood sugar levels, and other health parameters is important for tracking progress and making necessary adjustments to the weight management plan.

   - Working with a healthcare provider or registered dietitian who specializes in diabetes care can provide valuable guidance and support for weight management.

Strategies for Weight Loss and Weight Maintenance

Weight management is an important aspect of diabetes care, as excess weight can contribute to insulin resistance and increase the risk of complications. For individuals with diabetes who are overweight or obese, the following strategies can help with weight loss and weight maintenance:

1. Set Realistic Goals:

   - Set achievable and realistic weight loss goals based on your current weight, health status, and lifestyle. Aim for gradual weight loss of about 1-2 pounds per week, as rapid weight loss can be difficult to sustain and may not be healthy.

2. Create a Calorie Deficit:

   - To lose weight, you need to create a calorie deficit by consuming fewer calories than your body needs for maintenance. This can be achieved through a combination of dietary changes and increased physical activity.

3. Focus on Nutrition:

   - Emphasize nutrient-dense foods that are low in calories but high in essential nutrients, such as fruits, vegetables, whole grains, lean proteins, and healthy fats. These foods can help you feel full and satisfied while providing important vitamins and minerals.

4. Portion Control:

   - Be mindful of portion sizes and avoid overeating. Use smaller plates and utensils to help control portion sizes, and pay attention to serving sizes listed on food labels.

5. Monitor Your Intake:

   - Keep a food diary to track your daily food intake, including portion sizes and calorie counts. This can help you identify eating patterns, track your progress, and make adjustments as needed.

6. Limit Sugary Foods and Beverages:

   - Sugary foods and beverages can contribute to weight gain and cause rapid spikes in blood sugar levels. Limit your intake of sugary treats, sodas, fruit juices, and other high-calorie, high-sugar foods.

7. Be Active:

   - Incorporate regular physical activity into your routine to help burn calories and improve overall health. Aim for at least 150 minutes of moderate-intensity aerobic activity per week, along with muscle-strengthening activities on two or more days per week.

8. Seek Support:

   - Consider joining a weight loss program or working with a healthcare provider, dietitian, or certified diabetes educator to develop a personalized weight loss plan. Having support and guidance can increase your chances of success.

9. Monitor Your Progress:

   - Regularly monitor your weight, body measurements, and progress towards your weight loss goals. Celebrate your successes and make adjustments to your plan as needed to stay on track.

10. Maintain a Healthy Lifestyle:
  - Once you've achieved your weight loss goals, focus on maintaining a healthy lifestyle that includes a balanced diet, regular physical activity, and ongoing support to prevent weight regain.

Exercise and Its Impact on Blood Sugar and Weight

Exercise is a crucial component of diabetes management, offering numerous benefits for both blood sugar control and weight management. Here's a look at how exercise can impact blood sugar levels and weight in individuals with diabetes:

1. Blood Sugar Control:
  - Physical activity can help lower blood sugar levels by increasing the body's sensitivity to insulin. During exercise, muscles use glucose for energy, which can help reduce excess glucose in the bloodstream.

- Regular physical activity can improve insulin sensitivity, allowing the body to use insulin more effectively to lower blood sugar levels. This can be especially beneficial for individuals with insulin resistance, a common feature of type 2 diabetes.
- Exercise can also contribute to better overall blood sugar management by promoting weight loss, which can in turn improve insulin sensitivity and glycemic control.

2. Weight Management:
- Exercise plays a key role in weight management by helping individuals achieve and maintain a healthy weight. Being overweight or obese is a risk factor for type 2 diabetes and can worsen insulin resistance.
- Regular physical activity can help individuals with diabetes achieve weight loss goals by burning calories and increasing metabolism. Combining exercise with a healthy diet is often the most effective approach to weight management.

3. Types of Exercise:
- Aerobic Exercise: Activities like walking, cycling, swimming, and dancing are examples of aerobic exercise that can help improve cardiovascular health and contribute to weight management.

- Strength Training: Resistance training, using weights or resistance bands, can help build muscle mass, which can increase metabolism and improve overall body composition.

- Flexibility and Balance Exercises: Yoga, tai chi, and stretching exercises can improve flexibility, balance, and overall mobility, which can be beneficial for individuals with diabetes who may be at risk of falls or other complications.

4. Exercise Guidelines:

- Aim for at least 150 minutes of moderate-intensity aerobic exercise per week, spread out over at least three days, with no more than two consecutive days without activity.

- Incorporate strength training exercises at least two days per week, targeting major muscle groups.

- Always consult with a healthcare provider before starting a new exercise program, especially if you have any existing health conditions or concerns.

5. Monitoring Blood Sugar During Exercise:

- Monitor your blood sugar levels before, during, and after exercise to understand how physical activity affects your body. Adjust your diabetes management

plan as needed based on your blood sugar readings
and how you feel during exercise.

75

Chapter 8: Meal Prep and Cooking Tips for Diabetes

Meal Planning and Grocery Shopping Tips

Meal planning and smart grocery shopping are essential components of a diabetes-friendly diet. By carefully selecting ingredients and planning meals ahead of time, individuals with diabetes can make healthier choices and better manage their blood sugar levels. Here are some meal planning and grocery shopping tips for diabetes:

1. Plan Meals in Advance:
   - Take time to plan your meals for the week, considering a balance of carbohydrates, proteins, fats,

and fiber. Aim for variety and include a mix of different food groups.

   - Consider your schedule and lifestyle when planning meals. Choose recipes that are practical and achievable based on your available time and cooking skills.

2. Create a Shopping List:

   - Based on your meal plan, create a shopping list of the ingredients you'll need for the week. Organize your list by food categories (e.g., produce, dairy, proteins) to make shopping more efficient.

   - Stick to your list while shopping to avoid impulse purchases and ensure you have everything you need for your planned meals.

3. Choose Whole Foods:

   - Focus on whole, unprocessed foods when planning your meals and shopping. These include fruits, vegetables, whole grains, lean proteins, and healthy fats.

   - Minimize the use of processed foods, which often contain added sugars, unhealthy fats, and preservatives that can negatively impact blood sugar levels.

4. Read Food Labels:

   - When selecting packaged foods, carefully read food labels to check for the carbohydrate content, added sugars, and serving sizes. Choose products with lower sugar and sodium content.

   - Pay attention to portion sizes to ensure you're consuming appropriate amounts of carbohydrates and other nutrients.

5. Shop the Perimeter of the Store:

   - The perimeter of the grocery store typically contains fresh produce, meats, dairy, and other whole foods. Try to focus your shopping on these areas to fill your cart with nutritious options.

6. Consider Frozen and Canned Options:

   - Frozen fruits and vegetables can be convenient alternatives to fresh produce and are often just as nutritious. Look for options without added sugars or sauces.

   - Canned goods like beans, tomatoes, and fish can also be healthy additions to your pantry, but choose options with no added sugars or excess sodium.

7. Be Mindful of Portions:

- Consider portion sizes when purchasing foods. Buy single-serving packages or portion out larger quantities at home to avoid overeating.

8. Avoid Shopping When Hungry:
- Shopping on an empty stomach can lead to impulse purchases of unhealthy foods. Eat a balanced meal or snack before shopping to help you make better choices.

Cooking Methods for Diabetes-Friendly Meals

Choosing the right cooking methods is crucial for preparing diabetes-friendly meals that are both nutritious and flavorful. Here are some cooking methods that can help you create delicious and healthy meals while managing your blood sugar levels:

1. Grilling: Grilling is a great way to cook lean proteins like chicken, fish, and vegetables without adding extra fat. Use marinades with herbs, spices, and citrus juices

to add flavor without increasing the calorie or carbohydrate content.

2. Baking and Roasting: Baking and roasting are healthy cooking methods that require little to no added fat. You can bake or roast a variety of foods, including meats, poultry, fish, and vegetables, using herbs and spices for flavor.

3. Steaming: Steaming is a gentle cooking method that helps retain the nutrients in foods. Use a steamer basket or microwave steamer to steam vegetables, fish, and other foods without adding oil or butter.

4. Stir-Frying: Stir-frying involves quickly cooking small pieces of food in a small amount of oil over high heat. Use heart-healthy oils like olive or canola oil and plenty of vegetables to create flavorful stir-fries.

5. Sautéing: Sautéing is similar to stir-frying but uses less oil and lower heat. Use a non-stick pan and a small amount of oil to sauté vegetables, lean meats, or tofu.

6. Slow Cooking: Slow cooking is a convenient method for preparing meals ahead of time. Use a slow cooker

to cook soups, stews, and casseroles with lean proteins, whole grains, and plenty of vegetables.

7. Griddling: Griddling involves cooking foods on a flat, heated surface, such as a griddle or non-stick pan. It's a versatile method for cooking foods like pancakes, eggs, and sandwiches without added fat.

8. Poaching: Poaching involves gently cooking foods in liquid, such as water or broth, at a low temperature. Poaching is a healthy method for cooking fish, chicken, and eggs.

9. Microwaving: Microwaving is a quick and convenient cooking method that requires little to no added fat. Use microwave-safe containers to cook vegetables, grains, and proteins with minimal added oil or butter.

10. Healthy Oil Choices: When using oil for cooking, choose heart-healthy options like olive oil, canola oil, or avocado oil. Use them sparingly to control calorie and fat intake.

Chapter 9: Dining Out and Traveling with Diabetes

Tips for Dining Out with Diabetes

Dining out can be enjoyable and manageable for individuals with diabetes with some planning and awareness. Here are some tips for dining out with diabetes:

1. Research the Restaurant:
   - Choose restaurants that offer a variety of healthy options, such as grilled proteins, salads, and vegetable sides.
   - Look for nutrition information online or call the restaurant ahead of time to inquire about menu items that fit your dietary needs.

2. Plan Your Meal:

   - Review the menu and select a meal that includes a balance of carbohydrates, proteins, and fats.

   - Consider how the meal will affect your blood sugar levels and make adjustments to your insulin or medication as needed.

3. Watch Portion Sizes:

   - Be mindful of portion sizes, which can be larger than necessary in restaurants.

   - Consider sharing a meal with a dining companion or asking for a half-portion if available.

4. Be Mindful of Carbohydrates:

   - Choose carbohydrate-rich foods in moderation and be aware of hidden sugars in sauces, dressings, and marinades.

   - Opt for whole grains and fiber-rich foods when available to help manage blood sugar levels.

5. Monitor Alcohol Intake:

   - If you choose to drink alcohol, do so in moderation and with food to avoid hypoglycemia.

   - Be aware of the carbohydrate content and potential impact on blood sugar levels of alcoholic beverages.

6. Ask Questions:

   - Don't hesitate to ask your server about how dishes are prepared and whether modifications can be made to accommodate your dietary needs.
   - Request sauces and dressings on the side to control your intake of added sugars and fats.

7. Be Prepared:

   - Bring diabetes supplies such as glucose monitoring devices, insulin, and snacks in case of unexpected delays or changes in your meal plan.
   - Inform your dining companions about your dietary needs and how they can support you during the meal.

8. Stay Active:

   - If possible, engage in physical activity before or after your meal to help manage blood sugar levels.
   - Consider taking a walk after dining to aid digestion and regulate blood sugar.

9. Enjoy in Moderation:

   - While it's important to make healthy choices, it's also okay to enjoy a treat occasionally.
   - Be mindful of your overall dietary balance and make adjustments as needed in subsequent meals.

Remember to listen to your body and make adjustments based on how different foods and meals affect you individually.

Managing Diabetes While Traveling

Traveling can present unique challenges for individuals with diabetes, but with careful planning and preparation, it's possible to manage your condition effectively while on the go. Here are some tips for managing diabetes while traveling:

1. Plan Ahead:
   - Before your trip, consult with your healthcare provider to ensure that your diabetes management plan is up to date. Discuss any adjustments to your medication schedule, especially if you're traveling across time zones.
   - Pack all necessary diabetes supplies, including medications, insulin (if applicable), blood glucose monitoring supplies, snacks for low blood sugar, and a glucagon emergency kit if prescribed.

2. Keep Medications and Supplies Handy:

  - Carry your medications and supplies in your carry-on bag when flying or in a easily accessible bag when traveling by other means. This ensures that you have access to them at all times, even if your checked luggage is delayed or lost.

  - If you're traveling internationally, be aware of any restrictions on bringing medications and supplies into your destination country. Some countries may have specific regulations or require documentation for certain medications.

3. Monitor Blood Sugar Levels:

  - Check your blood sugar levels regularly, especially if your routine is disrupted by travel. Changes in diet, activity levels, and time zones can all affect your blood sugar levels.

  - Keep a record of your blood sugar readings and any adjustments you make to your diabetes management plan while traveling. This can help you track patterns and make informed decisions about your care.

4. Stay Hydrated and Eat Regularly:

- Drink plenty of water to stay hydrated, especially if you're flying or visiting a warmer climate. Dehydration can affect blood sugar levels and overall well-being.

- Stick to your regular meal schedule as much as possible. If your travel plans disrupt your usual meal times, carry healthy snacks with you to prevent low blood sugar.

5. Be Prepared for Emergencies:

- Familiarize yourself with the local healthcare resources at your destination, including the location of hospitals, clinics, and pharmacies.

- Carry a form of identification that indicates you have diabetes, such as a medical alert bracelet or card. This can be crucial in case of a medical emergency.

6. Communicate with Travel Companions:

- If you're traveling with others, make sure they are aware of your diabetes and how to help in case of an emergency.

- Educate your travel companions about the signs and symptoms of low and high blood sugar levels, as well as how to administer glucagon if necessary.

7. Manage Stress and Rest:

- Traveling can be stressful, which can affect blood sugar levels. Practice stress-reducing techniques such as deep breathing, meditation, or yoga to help manage stress.

- Get adequate rest and prioritize sleep, especially if you're traveling across time zones. Lack of sleep can affect blood sugar control and overall well-being.

Chapter 10: Monitoring and Adjusting Your Diet

Monitoring Blood Sugar Levels

Monitoring your blood sugar levels is a crucial part of managing diabetes and can provide valuable insights into how your body responds to different foods, activities, and medications. Here are some tips for monitoring your blood sugar levels effectively:

Establish a Monitoring Schedule:

Work with your healthcare provider to establish a monitoring schedule that meets your individual needs. This may include checking your blood sugar levels at specific times of the day, such as before meals, after meals, before bedtime, or during physical activity.

Your healthcare provider may recommend more frequent monitoring during times of illness, stress, or when there are changes to your diabetes management plan.

Use a Blood Glucose Meter:

A glucometer, also known as a blood glucose meter, is a portable device used to measure the concentration of glucose (sugar) in a drop of blood. It's an essential tool for individuals with diabetes, as it allows them to monitor their blood sugar levels regularly at home or on the go. Here's an extensive overview of glucometers and the values for normal and high blood sugar levels:

 How Glucometers Work:
- Glucometers typically use a small lancet to prick the skin and obtain a drop of blood, which is then placed on a test strip.
- The test strip contains enzymes that react with the glucose in the blood, producing a small electrical current.

- The meter measures this current and converts it into a digital display of the blood glucose level, usually in milligrams per deciliter (mg/dL) or millimoles per liter (mmol/L).

Normal Blood Sugar Levels:
- For individuals without diabetes, normal fasting blood sugar levels are typically between 70 to 99 mg/dL (3.9 to 5.5 mmol/L).
- After meals (postprandial), blood sugar levels in non-diabetic individuals may rise temporarily, but they usually return to normal levels within a few hours.

High Blood Sugar Levels (Hyperglycemia):
- Blood sugar levels above the normal range can indicate hyperglycemia, which is a common concern for people with diabetes.
- The threshold for diagnosing hyperglycemia varies, but generally, fasting blood sugar levels above 126 mg/dL (7.0 mmol/L) on two separate occasions are considered indicative of diabetes.
- After-meal blood sugar levels that consistently exceed 180 mg/dL (10.0 mmol/L) may also indicate poorly controlled diabetes.

Importance of Monitoring:

- Regular monitoring of blood sugar levels with a glucometer is crucial for individuals with diabetes to track their glucose control.
- It helps them understand how their diet, physical activity, medications, and other factors affect their blood sugar levels.
- Monitoring also allows for timely adjustments to diabetes management plans, such as medication dosages, meal planning, and lifestyle modifications.

 Using Glucometer Readings for Decision-Making:
- Glucometer readings guide important decisions in diabetes management, such as adjusting insulin doses, choosing appropriate foods, and recognizing and treating episodes of hypoglycemia (low blood sugar) or hyperglycemia.
- Target blood sugar ranges can vary based on individual factors such as age, type of diabetes, overall health, and treatment goals. Your healthcare provider can help you determine your specific targets.

Technology Advancements:
- Glucometer technology has advanced in recent years, with many devices offering features such as Bluetooth connectivity for data sharing with smartphones or cloud storage, alternative site testing

(AST) for blood collection from areas other than the fingertip, and the ability to store a large number of readings for long-term tracking.

 Accuracy and Calibration:
- Accuracy is a critical factor for glucometers, and manufacturers must ensure that their devices meet strict accuracy standards set by regulatory agencies.
- Regular calibration and quality control checks are important to ensure the accuracy of the readings. Users should follow the manufacturer's instructions for proper use and maintenance of the glucometer.

Working with a Healthcare Team

Managing your diet effectively with diabetes often requires collaboration with a healthcare team consisting of various professionals who can provide guidance and support. Here's how you can work with your healthcare team to monitor and adjust your diet:

1. Registered Dietitian or Nutritionist:

- A registered dietitian or nutritionist can help you develop a personalized meal plan based on your dietary needs, lifestyle, and health goals.

- Work with your dietitian to understand how different foods affect your blood sugar levels and how to make healthy choices that align with your diabetes management plan.

- Regularly review your meal plan with your dietitian to make adjustments as needed based on changes in your health status or dietary preferences.

2. Endocrinologist or Primary Care Physician:

- Your endocrinologist or primary care physician plays a key role in managing your overall diabetes care, including monitoring your blood sugar levels, prescribing medications, and addressing any concerns related to your diet.

- Keep your healthcare team informed about any changes in your diet, lifestyle, or health status that may impact your diabetes management. This includes changes in your weight, physical activity level, or the introduction of new foods or dietary supplements.

3. Certified Diabetes Educator (CDE):

- A certified diabetes educator can provide education and support related to diabetes self-management, including meal planning, blood sugar monitoring, and medication management.

   - Work with your CDE to develop practical strategies for managing your diet in real-life situations, such as dining out, traveling, or dealing with special occasions.

4. Other Healthcare Professionals:

   - Depending on your individual needs, you may also work with other healthcare professionals such as a pharmacist, psychologist, or exercise physiologist as part of your diabetes care team.

   - These professionals can provide additional support and expertise in areas such as medication management, mental health, and physical activity, all of which can impact your dietary choices and overall well-being.

5. Communication and Collaboration:

   - Effective communication with your healthcare team is essential for successful diabetes management. Keep your healthcare team informed about your dietary habits, challenges, and successes.

   - Be proactive in seeking guidance and asking questions about your diet and diabetes management. Take advantage of regular appointments to discuss any concerns or questions you may have.

6. Regular Monitoring and Follow-Up:

   - Schedule regular appointments with your healthcare team to monitor your progress, review your diet and meal plan, and make any necessary adjustments.

   - Use these appointments as an opportunity to discuss any challenges you may be facing with your diet and to seek guidance on how to overcome them.

Dietary Plan For A Month

Week 1: Sample Diabetic Meal Plan

 Day 1
- Breakfast:
  - 1 small whole-grain bagel with 1 tablespoon of almond butter
  - 1 medium apple
  - Unsweetened herbal tea or black coffee

- Lunch:
  - Grilled chicken salad with mixed greens, cherry tomatoes, cucumbers, and a vinaigrette dressing

  - 1 small whole-grain roll

- Dinner:
  - Baked salmon with roasted vegetables (broccoli, cauliflower, carrots) tossed in olive oil and herbs
  - 1/2 cup quinoa or brown rice

- Snack:
  - 1/4 cup unsalted mixed nuts
  - 1 small orange

Day 2
- Breakfast:
  - Greek yogurt parfait with plain Greek yogurt, mixed berries, and a sprinkle of chia seeds
  - Whole-grain toast (1 slice)

- Lunch:
  - Turkey and avocado wrap made with whole-grain tortilla, lettuce, and tomato
  - Baby carrots with hummus

- Dinner:
  - Stir-fried tofu with mixed vegetables (bell peppers, snap peas, onions) in a light soy sauce
  - 1/2 cup cooked quinoa or brown rice

- Snack:
  - Celery sticks with almond butter

Day 3
- Breakfast:
  - Spinach and feta omelet
  - 1 slice of whole-grain toast

- Lunch:
  - Lentil soup with a side of mixed greens salad and vinaigrette dressing
  - Whole-grain crackers (5-6 pieces)

- Dinner:
  - Grilled shrimp skewers with zucchini and bell peppers
  - 1/2 cup cooked quinoa or brown rice

- Snack:
  - Sugar-free yogurt with a sprinkle of cinnamon

Day 4
- Breakfast:
  - Smoothie made with unsweetened almond milk, spinach, frozen berries, and a scoop of protein powder

  - 1 hard-boiled egg

- Lunch:
  - Chicken Caesar salad with grilled chicken breast, romaine lettuce, Parmesan cheese, and Caesar dressing
  - 1 small whole-grain roll

- Dinner:
  - Baked cod fillet with steamed broccoli and a side of roasted sweet potatoes
  - Mixed berries for dessert

- Snack:
  - Raw veggies (carrots, bell peppers) with hummus

Day 5
- Breakfast:
  - Overnight oats made with rolled oats, unsweetened almond milk, chia seeds, and topped with sliced almonds and berries

- Lunch:
  - Quinoa salad with mixed vegetables, chickpeas, and a lemon-tahini dressing
  - 1 small orange

- Dinner:
  - Grilled chicken breast with asparagus and a side of wild rice
  - Mixed nuts for dessert

- Snack:
  - Apple slices with almond butter

Day 6
- Breakfast:
  - Whole-grain waffle with Greek yogurt and mixed berries
  - Black coffee or herbal tea

- Lunch:
  - Turkey and cheese sandwich on whole-grain bread with lettuce, tomato, and mustard
  - Carrot sticks with hummus

- Dinner:
  - Beef stir-fry with mixed vegetables in a light soy sauce
  - 1/2 cup cooked quinoa or brown rice

- Snack:

- Sugar-free pudding cup

Day 7
- Breakfast:
  - Scrambled eggs with spinach and tomatoes
  - Whole-grain toast (1 slice)

- Lunch:
  - Tuna salad made with canned tuna, mixed greens, cherry tomatoes, and a vinaigrette dressing
  - Whole-grain crackers (5-6 pieces)

- Dinner:
  - Grilled salmon with a side of steamed green beans and quinoa
  - Mixed berries for dessert

- Snack:
  - Greek yogurt with a sprinkle of cinnamon

Week 2: Sample Diabetic Meal Plan

Day 8
- Breakfast:
  - Spinach and mushroom omelet
  - Whole-grain toast (1 slice)

- Lunch:
  - Quinoa and black bean salad with diced tomatoes, bell peppers, and a lime-cilantro dressing
  - Sugar-free gelatin for dessert

- Dinner:
  - Grilled chicken breast with a side of steamed broccoli and cauliflower
  - 1/2 cup cooked wild rice

- Snack:
  - Cottage cheese with pineapple chunks

Day 9
- Breakfast:
  - Greek yogurt with sliced almonds and a drizzle of honey
  - Whole-grain toast (1 slice)

- Lunch:
  - Turkey and avocado wrap made with whole-grain tortilla, lettuce, and tomato
  - Baby carrots with hummus

- Dinner:

- Baked cod fillet with roasted Brussels sprouts and a side of quinoa
  - Mixed berries for dessert

- Snack:
  - Handful of walnuts

Day 10
- Breakfast:
  - Smoothie made with unsweetened almond milk, spinach, banana, and a scoop of protein powder
  - 1 hard-boiled egg

- Lunch:
  - Lentil soup with a side of mixed greens salad and vinaigrette dressing
  - Whole-grain crackers (5-6 pieces)

- Dinner:
  - Grilled shrimp skewers with zucchini and bell peppers
  - 1/2 cup cooked quinoa or brown rice

- Snack:
  - Sugar-free yogurt with a sprinkle of cinnamon

Day 11
- Breakfast:
  - Whole-grain oatmeal with sliced strawberries and a sprinkle of chia seeds
  - Black coffee or herbal tea

- Lunch:
  - Chicken Caesar salad with grilled chicken breast, romaine lettuce, Parmesan cheese, and Caesar dressing
  - 1 small whole-grain roll

- Dinner:
  - Stir-fried tofu with mixed vegetables (bell peppers, snap peas, onions) in a light soy sauce
  - 1/2 cup cooked quinoa or brown rice

- Snack:
  - Celery sticks with almond butter

Day 12
- Breakfast:
  - Whole-grain waffle with Greek yogurt and mixed berries
  - Black coffee or herbal tea

- Lunch:
  - Turkey and cheese sandwich on whole-grain bread
with lettuce, tomato, and mustard
  - Carrot sticks with hummus

- Dinner:
  - Beef stir-fry with mixed vegetables in a light soy
sauce
  - 1/2 cup cooked quinoa or brown rice

- Snack:
  - Apple slices with almond butter

 Day 13
- Breakfast:
  - Scrambled eggs with spinach and tomatoes
  - Whole-grain toast (1 slice)

- Lunch:
  - Tuna salad made with canned tuna, mixed greens,
cherry tomatoes, and a vinaigrette dressing
   Whole-grain crackers (5-6 pieces)

- Dinner:
  - Grilled salmon with a side of steamed green beans
and quinoa

  - Mixed berries for dessert

- Snack:
  - Greek yogurt with a sprinkle of cinnamon

 Day 14
- Breakfast:
  - Overnight oats made with rolled oats, unsweetened almond milk, chia seeds, and topped with sliced almonds and berries

- Lunch:
  - Turkey and avocado wrap made with whole-grain tortilla, lettuce, and tomato
  - Baby carrots with hummus

- Dinner:
  - Baked chicken breast with roasted vegetables (bell peppers, zucchini, onions) tossed in olive oil and herbs
  - 1/2 cup cooked quinoa or brown rice

- Snack:
  - Sugar-free pudding cup

Week 3: Sample Diabetic Meal Plan

Day 15
- Breakfast:
  - Whole-grain toast with avocado spread and a poached egg
  - Black coffee or herbal tea

- Lunch:
  - Grilled chicken salad with mixed greens, cherry tomatoes, cucumbers, and a vinaigrette dressing
  - 1 small whole-grain roll

- Dinner:
  - Baked salmon with roasted vegetables (asparagus, bell peppers, onions) tossed in olive oil and herbs
  - 1/2 cup quinoa or brown rice

- Snack:
  - 1/4 cup unsalted mixed nuts
  - 1 small orange

Day 16
- Breakfast:
  - Greek yogurt parfait with plain Greek yogurt, mixed berries, and a sprinkle of granola
  - Whole-grain toast (1 slice)

- Lunch:
  - Turkey and cheese sandwich on whole-grain bread with lettuce, tomato, and mustard
  - Baby carrots with hummus

- Dinner:
  - Stir-fried tofu with mixed vegetables (broccoli, snap peas, carrots) in a light soy sauce
  - 1/2 cup cooked quinoa or brown rice

- Snack:
  - Celery sticks with almond butter

Day 17
- Breakfast:
  - Spinach and feta omelet
  - Whole-grain toast (1 slice)

- Lunch:
  - Lentil soup with a side of mixed greens salad and vinaigrette dressing
  - Whole-grain crackers (5-6 pieces)

- Dinner:
  - Grilled shrimp skewers with zucchini and cherry tomatoes

 - 1/2 cup cooked quinoa or brown rice

- Snack:
 - Sugar-free yogurt with a sprinkle of cinnamon

Day 18
- Breakfast:
 - Smoothie made with unsweetened almond milk,
spinach, frozen berries, and a scoop of protein powder
 - 1 hard-boiled egg

- Lunch:
 - Chicken Caesar salad with grilled chicken breast,
romaine lettuce, Parmesan cheese, and Caesar
dressing
 - 1 small whole-grain roll

- Dinner:
 - Baked cod fillet with steamed broccoli and a side of
wild rice
 - Mixed berries for dessert

- Snack:
 - Raw veggies (carrots, bell peppers) with hummus

Day 19

- Breakfast:
  - Whole-grain oatmeal with sliced strawberries and a sprinkle of chia seeds
  - Black coffee or herbal tea

- Lunch:
  - Turkey and cheese wrap with lettuce, tomato, and whole-grain tortilla
  - Baby carrots with hummus

- Dinner:
  - Beef stir-fry with mixed vegetables in a light soy sauce
  - 1/2 cup cooked quinoa or brown rice

- Snack:
  - Apple slices with almond butter

Day 20
- Breakfast:
  - Whole-grain waffle with Greek yogurt and mixed berries
  - Black coffee or herbal tea

- Lunch:

- Tuna salad made with canned tuna, mixed greens, cherry tomatoes, and a vinaigrette dressing
  - Whole-grain crackers (5-6 pieces)

- Dinner:
  - Grilled salmon with a side of steamed green beans and quinoa
  - Mixed berries for dessert

- Snack:
  - Greek yogurt with a sprinkle of cinnamon

Day 21
- Breakfast:
  - Overnight oats made with rolled oats, unsweetened almond milk, chia seeds, and topped with sliced almonds and berries

- Lunch:
  - Turkey and avocado wrap made with whole-grain tortilla, lettuce, and tomato
  - Baby carrots with hummus

- Dinner:
  - Baked chicken breast with roasted vegetables (bell peppers, zucchini, onions) tossed in olive oil and herbs

  - 1/2 cup cooked quinoa or brown rice

- Snack:
  - Sugar-free pudding cup

Week 4: Sample Diabetic Meal Plan

Day 22
- Breakfast:
  - Scrambled eggs with spinach and tomatoes
  - Whole-grain toast (1 slice)

- Lunch:
  - Tuna salad made with canned tuna, mixed greens, cherry tomatoes, and a vinaigrette dressing
  - Whole-grain crackers (5-6 pieces)

- Dinner:
  - Grilled salmon with a side of steamed green beans and quinoa
  - Mixed berries for dessert

- Snack:
  - Greek yogurt with a sprinkle of cinnamon

Day 23

- Breakfast:
  - Overnight oats made with rolled oats, unsweetened almond milk, chia seeds, and topped with sliced almonds and berries

- Lunch:
  - Turkey and avocado wrap made with whole-grain tortilla, lettuce, and tomato
  - Baby carrots with hummus

- Dinner:
  - Baked chicken breast with roasted vegetables (bell peppers, zucchini, onions) tossed in olive oil and herbs
  - 1/2 cup cooked quinoa or brown rice

- Snack:
  - Sugar-free pudding cup

Day 24
- Breakfast:
  - Whole-grain waffle with Greek yogurt and mixed berries
  - Black coffee or herbal tea

- Lunch:

- Chicken Caesar salad with grilled chicken breast, romaine lettuce, Parmesan cheese, and Caesar dressing
  - 1 small whole-grain roll

- Dinner:
  - Stir-fried tofu with mixed vegetables (bell peppers, snap peas, onions) in a light soy sauce
  - 1/2 cup cooked quinoa or brown rice

- Snack:
  - Celery sticks with almond butter

Day 25
- Breakfast:
  - Smoothie made with unsweetened almond milk, spinach, banana, and a scoop of protein powder
  - 1 hard-boiled egg

- Lunch:
  - Lentil soup with a side of mixed greens salad and vinaigrette dressing
  - Whole-grain crackers (5-6 pieces)

- Dinner:

- Grilled shrimp skewers with zucchini and bell peppers
  - 1/2 cup cooked quinoa or brown rice

- Snack:
  - Sugar-free yogurt with a sprinkle of cinnamon

Day 26
- Breakfast:
  - Whole-grain oatmeal with sliced strawberries and a sprinkle of chia seeds
  - Black coffee or herbal tea

- Lunch:
  - Turkey and cheese sandwich on whole-grain bread with lettuce, tomato, and mustard
  - Carrot sticks with hummus

- Dinner:
  - Beef stir-fry with mixed vegetables in a light soy sauce
  - 1/2 cup cooked quinoa or brown rice

- Snack:
  - Apple slices with almond butter

Day 27
- Breakfast:
 - Greek yogurt with sliced almonds and a drizzle of
honey
 - Whole-grain toast (1 slice)

- Lunch:
 - Quinoa and black bean salad with diced tomatoes,
bell peppers, and a lime-cilantro dressing
 - Sugar-free gelatin for dessert

- Dinner:
 - Grilled chicken breast with a side of steamed
broccoli and cauliflower
 - 1/2 cup cooked wild rice

- Snack:
 - Cottage cheese with pineapple chunks

Day 28
- Breakfast:
 - Spinach and mushroom omelet
 - Whole-grain toast (1 slice)

- Lunch:

 - Quinoa salad with mixed vegetables, chickpeas, and a lemon-tahini dressing
   - 1 small orange

- Dinner:
 - Baked cod fillet with roasted Brussels sprouts and a side of quinoa
   - Mixed berries for dessert

- Snack:
  - Handful of walnuts

General Tips:
- Continue to focus on portion control and balanced meals.
- Monitor your blood sugar levels regularly and adjust your meals as needed.
- Stay hydrated by drinking plenty of water throughout the day.
- Incorporate a variety of foods to ensure you're getting essential nutrients.
- Be mindful of your carbohydrate intake and choose complex carbohydrates whenever possible.
- Aim for a mix of lean protein, healthy fats, and fiber-rich foods in your meals and snacks.

This plan is a sample and can be adjusted based on individual dietary needs, preferences, and any specific recommendations from a healthcare provider or dietitian.